A REPORT OF THE CSIS
GLOBAL HEALTH POLICY CENTER

Gaza's Health Sector under Hamas

INCURABLE ILLS?

Author
Haim Malka

February 2012

50 YEARS | CHARTING OUR FUTURE

CSIS | CENTER FOR STRATEGIC & INTERNATIONAL STUDIES

About CSIS—50th Anniversary Year

For 50 years, the Center for Strategic and International Studies (CSIS) has developed practical solutions to the world's greatest challenges. As we celebrate this milestone, CSIS scholars continue to provide strategic insights and bipartisan policy solutions to help decisionmakers chart a course toward a better world.

CSIS is a bipartisan, nonprofit organization headquartered in Washington, D.C. The Center's 220 full-time staff and large network of affiliated scholars conduct research and analysis and develop policy initiatives that look into the future and anticipate change.

Since 1962, CSIS has been dedicated to finding ways to sustain American prominence and prosperity as a force for good in the world. After 50 years, CSIS has become one of the world's preeminent international policy institutions focused on defense and security; regional stability; and transnational challenges ranging from energy and climate to global development and economic integration.

Former U.S. senator Sam Nunn has chaired the CSIS Board of Trustees since 1999. John J. Hamre became the Center's president and chief executive officer in 2000. CSIS was founded by David M. Abshire and Admiral Arleigh Burke.

CSIS does not take specific policy positions; accordingly, all views expressed herein should be understood to be solely those of the author(s).

Cover photo: A Hamas security forces officer walks inside a ward at the Shifa Hospital in Gaza City, August 9, 2007. Mohammed Abed/AFP/Getty Images.

ISBN: 978-089206-729-9 (pb)

Center for Strategic and International Studies
1800 K Street, NW, Washington, DC 20006
Tel: (202) 887-0200
Fax: (202) 775-3199
Web: www.csis.org

GAZA'S HEALTH SECTOR UNDER HAMAS

INCURABLE ILLS?

Haim Malka[1]

In less than three decades Hamas health care activities have transformed dramatically. This transformation in health care has mirrored Hamas's own evolution, albeit incomplete, from a militant organization to a de facto government. In the process the Islamic movement has gone from coordinating dozens of medical clinics and charities in the West Bank and Gaza to managing a multimillion dollar health ministry with thousands of employees and hundreds of thousands of beneficiaries. Once seen as a religious duty and a practical recruiting tool, Hamas's health care agenda is now one of practical governance and political survival.

Hamas's experience overseeing Gaza's government services has been both a challenge and an opportunity for the Islamic movement. Despite numerous setbacks, Gaza's health care sector under Hamas rule has remained remarkably resilient in the face of perpetual crisis. While it has ruled with a heavy hand, Hamas has proven its durability and resourcefulness. This predicament poses challenges for U.S. policy, which has sought to balance humanitarian support for Gaza's 1.6 million people while undermining Hamas and its violent ideology.

This paper traces the evolution of Hamas's health care services from the movement's origins to its current role as the de facto government of Gaza. The paper focuses primarily on the impact of Palestinian divisions on the development of Gaza's health sector since Hamas's takeover of Gaza in June 2007, and it examines how regional trends in 2011 have influenced internal Palestinian dynamics that will likely shape Gaza's health care sector and the Palestinian population more broadly in the future. Finally, the paper examines the U.S. policy implications of Hamas's successful management of health services in Gaza.[2]

---

[1] Haim Malka is a senior fellow and deputy director of the Middle East Program at the Center for Strategic and International Studies (CSIS) in Washington, DC.

[2] Though Israeli government policies, including restrictions on the flow of goods and people and the 2008–2009 Gaza War, undoubtedly affect Gaza's health care sector, that is a topic beyond the scope of this analysis. Numerous reports exist detailing the economic impact of Israel's closure policy and the Gaza War. See, for example, B'Tselem—The Israeli Information Center for Human Rights in the Occupied Territories, "The siege on the Gaza Strip: 1.5 million people imprisoned," May 31, 2010, http://www.btselem.org/gaza_strip/20100531_the_siege_on_gaza; and World Health Organization (WHO), "Report of the specialized health mission to the Gaza Strip," May 14, 2009, http://apps.who.int/gb/ebwha/pdf_files/A62/A62_24Add1-en.pdf.

Hamas Health Care Operations, Pre-June 2007

Social welfare and charity are core components of Hamas's ideology and have been central to the movement's popularity and success in establishing itself as an alternative to the secular-nationalist Fatah movement that dominated Palestinian politics for nearly four decades. Since September 11, 2001, Islamic charities and social service organizations have come under increasing scrutiny for connections to terrorist financing. While it is true that some charitable donations have gone to fund various terrorist organizations, including Hamas, the tradition of Islamic social welfare and charitable services has a centuries-long history.[3] The obligation of *zakat* or alms is considered one of the five pillars of Islamic faith and has provided the foundation for charitable enterprises that collect funds and distribute cash, food, and clothing to the needy.[4] In addition, Islamic charities provide a wide range of services including education, day care, health services, vocational training, and counseling.

When Hamas was established at the beginning of the First Intifada in 1987–1988, it essentially inherited the Muslim Brotherhood's existing network of social services and Islamic charities, which had been active for decades in the West Bank and Gaza. As Hamas grew in strength and popularity over the following decade it absorbed and exerted influence over numerous mosques, Islamic charities, and *zakat* committees, distributing aid to needy families and providing a range of social services.[5] By building an independent network of social services, as an alternative to the Israeli and Fatah systems, Hamas sought to form bonds with the Palestinian population that would later catapult the movement to the forefront of the Palestinian national movement.

More specifically, social services and charity played a crucial role in Hamas's activities and ideology in several ways.[6] First, social services, including education, were instrumental in Hamas's strategy to Islamize Palestinian society as a necessary precondition for creating an independent Palestinian state. Second, charities served to recruit and maintain networks of supporters that Hamas would later call on for social, political, and even military activity. Third, by building service networks

---

[3] For a comprehensive examination of Hamas charities before the 2007 Gaza takeover, see Haim Malka, "Hamas: Resistance and the Transformation of Palestinian Society," in *Understanding Islamic Charities*, ed. Jon B. Alterman and Karin Von Hippel (Washington, DC: CSIS, 2007), 98–126.

[4] *Zakat* is generally calculated as 2.5 percent of one's financial assets above a certain amount. There are specific formulas for calculating the amount of *zakat* a person should give based on income and assets. Shiite Muslims are usually required to give an additional portion of obligatory charity known as *khums* (one-fifth) on certain transactions and gains.

[5] *Zakat* committees are organizations that collect and distribute cash and in-kind donations. See, for example, Emanuel Schäublin, "The Role and Governance of Islamic Charitable Institutions: The West Bank Zakat Committees (1977–2009) in the Local Context," CCDP Working Paper No. 5, Graduate Institute of International and Development Studies, Geneva, November 2009, http://graduateinstitute.ch/webdav/site/ccdp/shared/6305/WP5_2_engl.pdf.

[6] For a more detailed analysis, see Malka, "Hamas: Resistance and Transformation of Palestinian Society," 105.

Hamas competed directly with the Palestinian Liberation Organization (PLO) and later the Palestinian Authority (PA) in providing services to the Palestinian population. Welfare has been Hamas's most effective form of activism. Unlike politics that often requires compromise and military operations that can elicit lethal reprisals, charity work is relatively risk free with high payoff.

It is difficult to assemble an accurate account of the magnitude of Hamas's social welfare network, but by 2003, it was estimated that one in six Palestinians received some form of support from Islamic social services organizations.[7] Examining the operations of Hamas affiliated institutions also provides insight into the scope of operations. One of Hamas's oldest social welfare organizations located in Gaza City, al-Mujamma al-Islami, for example, has an annual budget of nearly $1 million and 150 employees.

The center also operates over a dozen kindergartens and pays monthly stipends for nearly 5,000 orphans.[8] The Al Salah Association in southern Gaza, at one point reportedly operated four medical clinics that organization officials claimed served 15,000 people a month.[9] It also provided monthly support to the families of nearly 10,000 Palestinians who had lost their fathers, before its bank accounts were frozen in 2007.[10] In addition, *zakat* committees operate in nearly every Palestinian city, dispensing aid to the needy.

Hamas-affiliated charities and *zakat* committees are funded from a variety of sources. Inside the Palestinian Territories, Hamas depended on cash and in-kind donations from wealthy individuals, as well as from local business enterprises. Hamas has relied on aid from Iran for its political and military activity, while its affiliate charities were funded primarily by wealthy individuals and charitable organizations in the Gulf Arab states and Europe. According to one estimate published in 2006, international charities contributed $15 to $20 million a year to Hamas-linked charitable institutions.[11]

Hamas capitalized on these charities to build legitimacy and mobilize support. By providing badly needed services such as free primary health clinics, mobile clinics in rural areas, and funds for specialized treatments and operations, Hamas won over many poor and underprivileged

---

[7] International Crisis Group (ICG), "Islamic Social Welfare Activism in the Occupied Territories: A Legitimate Target?" ICG Middle East Report 13, International Crisis Group, Brussels, April 2, 2003, 12, http://www.crisisgroup.org/~/media/Files/Middle%20East%20North%20Africa/Israel%20Palestine/Islamic%20Social%20Welfare%20Activism%20In%20The%20Occupied%20Palestinian%20Territories.pdf.

[8] Ulrike Putz, "Uncle Hamas Cares for Palestinians," *Spiegel Online*, December 20, 2006, http://www.spiegel.de/international/0,1518,455632,00.html.

[9] Susan Taylor Martin, "Frozen Accounts Jeopardize Learning, Healing in Gaza," *St. Petersburg Times*, September 15, 2003, http://www.sptimes.com/2003/09/15/Worldandnation/Frozen_accounts_jeopa.shtml.

[10] Adam Entous, "U.S.-backed campaign against Hamas expands to charities," Reuters, August 20, 2007, http://www.reuters.com/article/2007/08/20/us-palestinians-hamas-idUSL2027514420070820.

[11] Matthew Levitt, *Hamas: Politics, Charity, and Terrorism in the Service of Jihad* (New Haven, CT: Yale University Press, 2006), 144.

Palestinians. Hamas would later exploit these bonds, occasionally to secure cover for military operations, but most importantly by deepening the dependence of many Palestinians on Hamas services during the 1990s.

At the same time, by providing basic services as well as privileged access to specialized and modern facilities, Hamas was able to strengthen its links with Palestinians of a similarly conservative and religious outlook. Fatah and the Palestinian Authority maintained health clinics reserved for PA employees or security personnel, the vast majority of whom were Fatah members. By operating similar networks of its own, Hamas was able to recruit loyal employees and supporters, campaign workers, voters, and soldiers.

Collectively, Hamas's record of effective and professional social welfare activities strengthened the movement's legitimacy and appeal among Palestinians and contributed to its electoral victory in 2006. That victory was a major turning point for the organization and ushered in new complications for the health care sector.

Hamas Health Care Operations, Post-June 2007

For most of its existence Hamas's health care networks largely coexisted with the Fatah-dominated and PA-run Ministry of Health (MoH) in both the West Bank and Gaza, as well as with international service providers such as the UN Relief and Works Agency (UNRWA). That coexistence became increasingly difficult to maintain after Hamas's election victory and the establishment of its first government in 2006. Despite efforts to form a unity government in March 2007, internal Palestinian divisions reemerged quickly.[12] In June 2007, months of tension and skirmishes erupted into open warfare. In a matter of days, Hamas forces seized all PA and Fatah security installations and government buildings and expelled Fatah's leadership. Over 100 people were killed and 500 left wounded.[13] The bloody takeover of Gaza was a watershed event, resulting in two de facto governments in Ramallah and Gaza with parallel Ministries of Health.

Egypt and Israel responded by sealing Gaza's borders, which deepened Hamas's international isolation, and further strained social services and health care. Hamas's health care network in Gaza

---

[12] Following its election victory in January 2006, Hamas formed its first government headed by Prime Minister Ismail Haniyeh. In March 2007, Hamas and Fatah formed a short-lived unity government following the Saudi sponsored Mecca Agreement.

[13] In the ensuing Hamas-Fatah clashes, hospitals and health care facilities not only treated hundreds of people wounded in the internal fighting, which left over 100 killed, but became the battleground for the Hamas-Fatah struggle in Gaza, as gun battles raged inside and near Palestinian hospitals. According to Human Rights Watch, Fatah gunmen fired mortars and rocket-propelled grenades at Shifa Hospital in Gaza City, drawing Hamas fire from inside the building, which killed one Hamas and one Fatah fighter. At a hospital in Beit Hanun, Hamas forces killed three family members with ties to Fatah and wounded others. See Human Rights Watch, "Gaza: Armed Palestinian Groups Commit Grave Crimes," June 12, 2007, http://www.hrw.org/en/news/2007/06/12/gaza-armed-palestinian-groups-commit-grave-crimes.

went from complementing and competing with existing PA services to bearing sole responsibility for overseeing health care for Gaza's 1.6 million people. Though Gaza benefitted from an influx of foreign development aid beginning in 1993, its health services have lagged compared to those of the West Bank. Rates of noncommunicable diseases and chronic disease are rising, while treatment remains limited.[14] Numerous reports also suggest that food security in Gaza has declined primarily in the quality of food people are consuming. When it took the reins of Gaza in mid-2007, Hamas inherited a health care infrastructure that was already strained and in danger of becoming more so.

Palestinian divisions have further politicized health care and reduced the quality and quantity of health care services available in Gaza. In response to Hamas's takeover of Gaza, the Ramallah PA arrested hundreds of Hamas activists and closed 132 Hamas-associated charities, effectively shutting down the movement's social services and charitable network in the West Bank.[15] A number of Hamas-affiliated health care facilities were also attacked.[16] Moreover, the Ramallah PA supported the Egyptian-Israeli closure of Gaza and manipulated the flow of medicine into Gaza in order to undermine and pressure the de facto Hamas government in the hope that it would collapse.[17]

Both governments in Gaza and Ramallah launched campaigns to fire public-sector employees affiliated with rival movements and promoted their own loyalists. In the health care sector, this included firing the administrators, directors, and boards of public hospitals, as well as physicians and nurses. A number of health sector strikes in the summer of 2007 and again in 2008 further crippled Gaza's health services. In another effort to undermine Hamas, the Ramallah PA cut the salaries of nearly 1,400 MoH employees affiliated with or appointed by Hamas and paid thousands of health care workers to refrain from working. The strikes effectively cut the number of health care workers in the public sector by as much as 60 percent of administrative staff and 40 percent of

---

[14] Gaza's infection rate for diseases associated with poor environmental health, for example, are considerably higher than in the West Bank. Acute hepatitis in Gaza (75.3 per 100,000) is high compared to the West Bank (15.9 per 100,000); typhoid fever is also high in Gaza (12.4 per 100,000) but nearly nonexistent in the West Bank (0.0 per 100,000). See WHO, "Health conditions in the occupied Palestinian territory, including east Jerusalem, and in the occupied Syrian Golan," May 13, 2010, http://unispal.un.org/UNISPAL.NSF/0/885BD85F892778F28525772700503A4B.

[15] The Ramallah PA froze the assets and closed 132 charitable organizations affiliated in varying degrees with Hamas. Of these 92 were *zakat* committees. See Schäublin, "The Role and Governance of Islamic Charitable Institutions."

[16] The Medical Scientific Society Center in Bediya (Salfit) was attacked and ransacked by PA security forces, and the Al Razi Hospital in Jenin was threatened with closure by the Fatah-linked Al Aksa Martyrs Brigade.

[17] See Donald Macintyre, "Palestinian power struggle swallows millions in aid cash," *The Independent*, November 5, 2008, accessed through Lexis-Nexus; and "Palestinian Health Ministry accuses West Bank government of withholding medicine," BBC Monitoring, August 8, 2011, accessed through Lexis-Nexis.

physicians and nurses. By 2009, Ramallah paid an estimated 7,000 health care workers, while the Hamas government paid another 2,000.[18]

Hamas, meanwhile, wasted no time in moving to consolidate its control over MoH, staffing many positions with its own loyalists, many of whom had less training and experience than the health care professionals they replaced. In some cases, Hamas used threats and intimidation to force doctors and nurses back to work, while also closing down private clinics run by Fatah loyalists—though Gaza's economic deterioration in the face of economic embargo, including its high rate of unemployment (estimated at over 40 percent in 2010),[19] was already shrinking the numbers of people who could afford care in private (for-profit) clinics and hospitals. The combination of these factors led to a decline in the quality of health care services available, as well as a decline in the supply of medicines and available services.

Hamas's shift from indirectly maintaining networks to directly administering services was colored by a much larger political process. While providing social services on such a large scale was a challenge, it was also an opportunity for Hamas to prove its administrative skills and creatively exploit various funding outlets.

Impressively, Hamas successfully balanced its immediate goal of preventing the collapse of the health sector with a broader restructuring of MoH, including the long-term goal of improving comprehensive health care services in Gaza. Today, those services form three tiers: clinics, which focus on vaccinations, prenatal care, chronic disease management, general medical consultations for children and adults, diagnostic services and dental care; secondary and referral services; and tertiary care for advanced and specialized issues.

According to the UN Development Programme (UNDP), the Hamas-run MoH oversees half of Gaza's 24 hospitals, which account for nearly 75 percent of all hospital beds, and 56 primary health clinics, or roughly half of health clinics.[20] The remaining hospitals are either private or administered by UNRWA. The most important source of funding for Gaza's services comes from the Ramallah-based PA, which uses tax revenues on goods and funds from the international donor community including the World Bank to pay salaries of PA employees in Gaza's Health, Social

---

[18] Are Hovdenak, ed., *The Public Services Under Hamas in Gaza: Islamic Revolution or Crisis Management?* PRIO Report 3-2010 (Oslo: Peace Research Institute Oslo, 2010), 23, http://www.prio.no/sptrans/873931406/The_Public_Services_under_Hamas_in_Gaza.pdf.

[19] See Salem Ajluni, "Labour Market Briefing: Gaza Strip: Second-half 2010," UN Relief and Works Agency (UNRWA), April 2011, http://www.unrwa.org/userfiles/201106083557.pdf. There are indications that Gaza's unemployment rate decreased in the first quarter of 2011 to as low as 31 percent. See Office of the UN Special Coordinator for the Middle East Peace Process, "Socio-economic Report: May 2011," http://www.unsco.org/Documents/Special/Socioeconomic%20Report%20May%202011.pdf.

[20] See WHO, "Health situation in Gaza—4 February 2009," http://www.who.int/hac/crises/international/wbgs/sitreps/gaza_4feb2009/en/; and UN Development Programme (UNDP), *One Year After Report: Gaza Early Recovery and Reconstruction Needs Assessment* (Jerusalem: UNDP, May 2010), http://www.undp.ps/en/newsroom/publications/pdf/other/gazaoneyear.pdf.

Affairs, and Education Ministries. These payments have been periodically delayed by the Ramallah PA. Ramallah-PA funds are also used to purchase fuel for the Gaza power plant and district water system.[21] The limited contact between the Gaza and Ramallah ministries is coordinated by Gaza MoH employees who are considered "loyalists" to the Ramallah PA and are paid by Ramallah.[22]

According to Hamas sources, as of July 2009, approximately 8,500 health staff worked in MoH facilities in Gaza. Nearly 6,500 are paid by the Ramallah PA, and the rest are paid by funds allocated by the Hamas government. There are reportedly an additional 2,000 trained health workers whom the Ramallah PA pays *not* to work. These include staff who went on strike in the second half of 2008 and whom Hamas had barred from returning to their jobs.[23]

The World Health Organization (WHO) estimates the 2010 PA MoH (Ramallah and Gaza combined) budget is approximately $354 million.[24] According to the Ramallah PA, 40 percent of the combined Gaza and Ramallah health budget should be allocated to the Gaza MoH by Ramallah. Still, there is no accurate figure available for the actual amount that Ramallah has transferred to the Gaza MoH.

More broadly, it is difficult to assemble a fully accurate accounting of Hamas's Gaza network, or the extent to which the Hamas movement funds Gaza government expenditures and vice versa. According to official Gaza PA figures, its 2010 budget was $540 million.[25] A portion of that revenue comes from taxes Hamas collects on goods smuggled through hundreds of tunnels between Gaza and the Egyptian Sinai.[26] Reports from Gaza suggest that Hamas collects approximately $42 to $48

---

[21] Al Jazeera, "Pay dispute closes Gaza power plant," August 7, 2010, http://www.aljazeera.com/news/middleeast/2010/08/20108792815777160.html. The European Union also contributes to an emergency water treatment project in Gaza. See European Union, "Drinking water in Gaza and rule of law: EU supports the PA in two focal sectors of intervention," press release, December 12, 2011, http://eeas.europa.eu/delegations/westbank/documents/news/20111212_water_ruleoflaw_agreements_en.pdf.

[22] Mahmoud ElMadhoun, "Case Study III: The Health Sector, in *The Public Services under Hamas in Gaza*, ed. Are Hovdenak, p. 67.

[23] WHO, "Gaza Health Assessment: July 2009," June 29, 2009, http://www.emro.who.int/palestine/reports%5Cmonitoring%5CWHO_special_monitoring%5Cgaza%5CGaza%20Health%20Assessment%20%2829Jun09%29.pdf.

[24] The total expenditure was 1,233 million new Israeli shekels (NIS). See WHO, "Health conditions in the occupied Palestinian territory, including east Jerusalem, and in the occupied Syrian Golan," May 17, 2011, http://apps.who.int/gb/ebwha/pdf_files/WHA64/A64_ID2-en.pdf.

[25] Mai Yaghi, "Hamas commercial ventures thrive in Gaza's besieged economy," *The Daily Star* (Beirut), July 26, 2010, http://www.dailystar.com.lb/Business/Middle-East/Jul/26/Hamas-commercial-ventures-thrive-in-Gazas-besieged-economy.ashx#axzz1gT5NqE5E.

[26] World Bank officials estimate that 80 percent of Gaza's imports came through the tunnels in 2009. Since then, easing Israeli restrictions have allowed more goods to cross between Israel and Gaza, which could lower tax revenues on smuggled goods. Erin Cunningham, "Hamas profits from Israel's Gaza blockade," *Christian Science Monitor*, August 17, 2009, http://www.csmonitor.com/World/Middle-East/2009/0817/p09s01-wome.html.

million a year through taxes on goods as well as other licensing fees.[27] It is widely believed that the vast majority of the remaining budget is contributed by foreign sources. Iran has been an important donor, though future funding may be in jeopardy following Hamas's departure from and impending break with the Bashar al-Assad regime in Syria, a key Iranian ally. Qatar has been another important source and reportedly has covered budget shortfalls by paying salaries in specific government ministries.[28]

In addition to the PA salary transfers, Gaza's health system benefits from nearly $200 million a year from UNRWA operations and nearly $98 million from various USAID projects, as well as donations from other international organizations operating in Gaza.[29] These organizations include local and international nongovernmental organizations (NGOs) and private for-profit providers, many of which operate health clinics and hospitals.[30] Hamas coordinates its own public health care services with this array of service providers, as well with international organizations such as the World Bank and WHO, which indirectly provide the vast majority of funding for Gaza's MoH.[31] Hamas also coordinates with numerous international and Islamic charities inside and outside of Gaza that provide additional medication, medical supplies, and other donations.

Hamas has skillfully harnessed all available funding and external support for maintaining services in Gaza. Without the payment of tens of thousands of salaries by the Ramallah PA, the local opposition to Hamas's government would be much greater; indeed, Ramallah's role in funding Gaza's health care and other services has been crucial to Hamas's survival, not only providing services but jobs. On a tactical level, Ramallah's funds have also given it the power to provide and withhold payments and medicines depending on the political environment. Ramallah has had to carefully balance its desire to use this power to undermine the Hamas government against creating a deeper crisis in Gaza's health services, which would worsen Gaza's economic crisis and erode the Ramallah leadership's claim to be the legitimate government of Palestinians. Lacking other recourse for funding, Hamas has had little choice but to accommodate this arrangement.

Thus, while Hamas is often credited with efficient bureaucratic management and competency, it could not have managed to administer Gaza's social services at the same level without the hundreds of millions of dollars it receives in foreign support. That support is crucial for covering the majority of its daily operations, including paying salaries, supplying medicine, and providing fuel and

---

[27] U.S. Consulate, Jerusalem, "Does Hamas Have a Cash Flow Problem in Gaza?" cable, February 12, 2010, http://www.cablegatesearch.net/cable.php?id=10JERUSALEM276.
[28] Ibid.
[29] The United States is the largest donor to UNRWA and contributed nearly $228 million from the beginning of FY2010 to August 2010, providing food, temporary shelter, and medical supplies. See Jim Zanotti, "U.S. Foreign Aid to the Palestinians," CRS Report, November 9, 2011, http://www.fas.org/sgp/crs/mideast/RS22967.pdf.
[30] Nidal al-Mughrabi, "U.S. suspends work of aid groups in Gaza Strip," Reuters, August 12, 2011, http://www.reuters.com/article/2011/08/13/us-palestinians-us-gaza-idUSTRE77C03Q20110813.
[31] Funding from the World Bank and WHO for the Gaza MoH is channeled through the Ramallah PA.

medical equipment. The Hamas government continues to benefit from this external support, despite ongoing efforts to isolate Hamas.

Amid constant turmoil, Gaza's health care has undergone a period of expansion. Hamas managed to increase the number of hospital beds in Gaza from approximately 1,500 in 2006 to 1,900 in 2008, as well as to double the number of beds in special care units to 30.[32] As part of its consolidation of the health care sector, Hamas appointed 2,500 new employees, including administrators, nurses, and physicians. The Gaza MoH also established the Palestinian Medical Board, which coordinates and oversees medical education and training. It has also attempted to streamline the budget by eliminating overtime and bonuses. In an effort to promote transparency and eliminate double salaries, all public-sector health care employees in Gaza must regularly provide bank statements to MoH before they can receive their salaries. More broadly, Hamas's management of the health care system has emphasized cost cutting and efficiency.

For all Hamas's skill at securing financial support for health care and improving administration, the challenges facing Gaza's health sector remain daunting. According to WHO, for example, in early January 2011 nearly 40 percent of essential drugs were out of stock in Gaza,[33] in part because of the Ramallah MoH's refusal to deliver them. (WHO officials estimate that the Ramallah-based PA provides nearly two-thirds of Gaza's pharmaceuticals, primarily using World Bank funds, with the Red Cross providing the majority of the rest.[34]) The Gaza MoH has purchased medicine on the local market, which is smuggled in via tunnels connected to the Egyptian Sinai, and also receives donations from international organizations via the Rafah crossing on the Egyptian border. However, the lack of donor coordination often results in oversupply of some medicines and undersupply of others.

Hamas has also occasionally sparred with international donors and aid groups working in Gaza. Though it benefits from this aid, coordination is complicated, and tension occasionally flares into crisis. In mid-2011, Hamas authorities escalated their surveillance and monitoring of foreign NGOs working in Gaza by demanding financial audits. At the time, the United States threatened to cut off nearly $100 million in humanitarian aid to Gaza if Hamas did not drop its demand to audit U.S. organizations operating there.[35] The episode was finally resolved, but demonstrates the precariousness of foreign aid operations in Gaza as well as Hamas's dependence on externally funded and operated humanitarian services.

---

[32] ElMadhoun, "Case Study III: The Health Sector," pp. 64–65.

[33] WHO, "Drug Shortages in Gaza: Background Note to the HC," February 3, 2011, http://www.lacs.ps/documentsShow.aspx?ATT_ID=3620.

[34] Tony Laurance, head of WHO's West Bank and Gaza office in Jerusalem, as reported in ElMadhoun, "Case Study III: The Health Sector," p. 64.

[35] Ethan Bronner, "U.S. Threatens to Halt Gaza Aid Over Hamas Audits, *New York Times*, August 11, 2011, http://www.nytimes.com/2011/08/12/world/middleeast/12gaza.html.

Another challenge is getting Gazans specialized medical care that is available only in Israel or abroad. This is a complex bureaucratic process involving permits from the Gaza MoH and the Ramallah MoH, as well as from several Israeli military bodies, including the Coordinator of Government Activities in the Territories (COGAT). The process is now managed by the Palestinian Referral Abroad Department, a highly politicized body, which Hamas accuses of consistently refusing referrals of patients sympathetic to Hamas. In mid-2009, Hamas and Fatah agreed to appoint an independent body to manage the Referral Department.

Hamas's broader approach to governance has also created difficulties for many Gazans. In securing its power and control of Gaza, Hamas resorted to increasingly authoritarian policies and restrictions, raising new challenges to its legitimacy among the population. Hamas authorities have limited freedom of speech and assembly by harassing and detaining civil society activists and peaceful demonstrators.[36] Moreover, it closely monitors government employees, creating an environment of intimidation, fear, and mistrust.[37]

Gaza's Political Future

Overall, the development of Gaza's health care sector has been part of a broader process that has forced Hamas to adapt to the policy needs of a government rather than merely the needs of a movement. As much as Hamas's political evolution and control of Gaza's government may unsettle Western observers, the process has sprung from the legitimate human security needs of Gaza's population and from contingencies of time, territory, and political allegiance that are outside the control of any single actor.

Yet Gaza's health care sector and the politics that structure it also do not exist in a vacuum. Regional uprisings and domestic pressures have created new demands on Hamas and its Palestinian rival Fatah to overcome their differences. A broad Palestinian convergence may emerge, shaped in part by the failure of Hamas and Fatah to achieve their respective basic goals. President Mahmoud Abbas of the Palestinian Authority appears to have given up on negotiating an agreement with the current Israeli government, while members of Hamas feel that the group can no longer isolate itself in Gaza while the rest of the region is changing. Leading members of both factions recognize that their deep divisions are a political liability and unpopular among the majority of Palestinians, and both have renewed efforts to reach a power-sharing arrangement that would restructure the PLO's leadership and pave the way for presidential and parliamentary elections.[38]

---

[36] Human Rights Watch, "Gaza: Stop Harassing Activists," August 22, 2011, http://www.hrw.org/news/2011/08/22/gaza-stop-harassing-activists.)

[37] Some reports have suggested that Hamas has attempted to segregate male and female employees in its health care centers and insist that its female employees dress according to conservative Islamic principles.

[38] On May 4, 2011, Hamas and Fatah representatives signed a broad power-sharing arrangement in Cairo that aimed to establish a unity government and set a date for legislative and presidential elections. The

A reconciliation process that leads to power sharing and cooperation between Hamas and Fatah could improve health care services for Palestinians (and social services more broadly) by depoliticizing the health infrastructure and increasing cooperation between Gaza and the West Bank. Over time, it could also de-link health care and other services from the partisan battle between Hamas and Fatah, paving the way for better quality, availability, and efficiency.

Despite the recent announcement of a unity government agreement signed in Doha, Qatar, tangible progress toward reconciliation that would end the political and geographical divisions between Hamas and Fatah are complicated by several factors.[39] First, Hamas's own internal political dynamics and competing priorities make strategic decisionmaking difficult. Second, powerful forces within both Palestinian factions are not eager to forgo their monopoly of control in their respective geographic entities. Broadly speaking, both Hamas and Fatah want to give the impression of progress, but ultimately they may not be ready to pay the price of an agreement that would solve the majority of their outstanding issues, most importantly control over security forces.

Still, Hamas seems well positioned to adapt to a changing strategic environment. Though its long-standing alliance with the Assad regime in Syria is collapsing, and ties with Iran are frayed, its broader regional prospects are improving. Egypt has moved from an adversary to a sympathetic partner and eased the blockade of Gaza imposed by the Hosni Mubarak regime. Turkey's AKP leadership has welcomed Hamas officials to Turkey and called for the reconstruction of Gaza. And Qatar is providing supplementary funding and political support. The wave of Islamist electoral victories across the region provides a more sympathetic regional political environment for Hamas, with greater Arab Sunni support as part of a broader Sunni effort to undermine Iran and its allies.

On the domestic front, Hamas scored a major political victory through the release of over 1,000 Palestinian prisoners in the October 2011 exchange deal with Israel.[40] And despite ongoing bouts of violence and Israeli threats of another military strike Gaza, Israel's security establishment largely recognizes that the status quo in Gaza is preferable to alternatives that could be much more destabilizing. Hamas will likely use these advantages to strengthen its domestic position, should elections move forward.

Regardless of whether Palestinian reconciliation evolves toward a workable power-sharing arrangement or whether the division intensifies, Hamas will remain actively involved in providing health care and other services to the Palestinian population in Gaza. If the Palestinian

---

negotiations were renewed in December 2011. For the text of the May agreement, see "Fateh and Hamas Reconciliation Agreement, May 4 2011," Jerusalem Media and Communications Center, http://www.jmcc.org/Documentsandmaps.aspx?id=828.

[39] Al Jazeera, "Abbas to head Palestinian unity government," February 6, 2012, http://www.aljazeera.com/news/middleeast/2012/02/20122610416298264.html.

[40] On October 18, 2011, Israel and Hamas exchanged Major Gilad Shalit of the Israeli Army, held in Hamas captivity since June 2006, for 477 Palestinian prisoners. Israel released the second round of 550 additional prisoners in December 2011.

reconciliation process advances, Hamas will likely seek to reconstitute and expand its activities in the West Bank, while maintaining a leading role in managing Gaza. Moreover, should Hamas formally join the PLO, it would give the movement another avenue to influence Palestinian communities living in refugee camps in Lebanon, Jordan, and Syria. In order to reach those communities, Hamas would have to revitalize the PLO, which withered as a result of the establishment of the PA, losing its connection to the Palestinian diaspora. Should the unity effort break down, however, Gaza will remain under full Hamas control, and health care will remain subject to the bitter struggle between Hamas and Fatah.

Though many Palestinians in Gaza are frustrated with Hamas's achievements and disillusioned by its authoritarian rule, there appears to be no practical alternative to its control of Gaza for the foreseeable future. Rather than the Ramallah PA regaining control over Gaza, a breakdown of Hamas authority, which is highly unlikely, would create a power vacuum that could be exploited by more radical forces and could lead to a flight of international donor organizations, ensuring a deterioration of services for Gaza's population.

At the same time, if the health care sector in Gaza is to reach its full potential, Hamas and Fatah must coordinate and cooperate more effectively, which includes moving toward a workable power-sharing arrangement. Greater cooperation is the most effective way to ensure the stability of Gaza's health sector, despite the political challenges of doing so. Beyond the health care sector, the success or failure of the reconciliation process will shape the broader Palestinian political context for the foreseeable future.

Ramifications for U.S. Policy

For the United States, the stakes of this process are both political and humanitarian. For nearly two decades, the U.S. government has worked with Palestinians who have renounced violence to create viable Palestinian institutions in preparation for Palestinian statehood, which the U.S. government has defined as a national interest.[41] A key, yet implicit, pillar of that policy has focused on weakening Hamas and supporting a nonviolent Palestinian alternative. The United States has spent nearly $4 billion in aid to the Fatah-led PA in the form of direct budgetary assistance, humanitarian aid, and security training toward those broader U.S. goals. U.S. efforts however, have been complicated by a commitment to providing humanitarian aid to Gaza without indirectly benefiting the Hamas government that rules Gaza. This has become an increasingly difficult balancing act, subject to intense scrutiny from U.S. lawmakers.

As the largest single contributor to UNRWA and WHO, the United States arguably relieves some of Hamas's burden for providing services to all of Gaza's citizens.[42] This has created friction between

---

[41] President of the United States, "National Security Strategy of the United States," White House, May 2010, http://www.whitehouse.gov/sites/default/files/rss_viewer/national_security_strategy.pdf.

[42] U.S. lawmakers have attempted to cut UNRWA funding, arguing that UNRWA employs Hamas sympathizers and activists and that Hamas siphons U.S. assistance.

the United States and UNRWA officials, who have consistently urged the United States and donor countries to cooperate with the Hamas authorities. Concerns that UNRWA cooperates with Hamas led to new understandings between the U.S. government and UNRWA in November 2010, which included a stricter vetting process for UNRWA employees and tracking of U.S. assistance funds.[43] The U.S. government has to carefully calibrate its support and navigate a maze of legal and political constraints. In the months ahead this balancing act will grow more complicated.

While the United States has supported President Abbas and the Ramallah PA with financial assistance and security training, Abbas has pursued independent policies, increasingly at odds with the U.S. approach. First, he has applied for full Palestinian UN membership status, disregarding the Obama administration's promise to veto any such vote in the Security Council. Having failed to achieve the necessary votes in the Security Council, Abbas has continued to seek full Palestinian membership in UN specialized agencies, such as UNESCO. A vote to admit Palestine as a full member state in late October 2011 triggered an automatic freeze on U.S. funding for UNESCO, which accounts for approximately 22 percent of the organization's budget.[44] Should the Palestinian leadership seek full membership in organizations such as WHO, it could have devastating consequences for the health of millions of people across the globe.

Second, should the Palestinian reconciliation process lead to a unity government, it would result in further U.S. funding cuts to the Palestinians. U.S. law prohibits funding a unity government that includes Hamas, and when Hamas and Fatah formed a unity government in March 2007, it prompted a freeze of U.S. funding. The law is more ambiguous when it comes to supporting a unity government composed of technocrats or ministers not directly affiliated with either Hamas or Fatah.[45] In either case, the prospect of a Palestinian unity government poses challenges for the U.S. government, and should the Palestinians move toward a power-sharing arrangement, it could intensify calls on Capitol Hill to cut Palestinian funding.

U.S. policy has thus far opposed Palestinian reconciliation as long as Hamas refuses to accept three conditions devised by the "Quartet" (the United States, the European Union, Russia, and the United Nations), namely: recognizing Israel, renouncing violence, and abiding by previous agreements signed between Israel and the PLO. Secretary of State Hillary Clinton recently reiterated U.S. opposition to such a unity government, claiming "We've made it very clear that we

---

[43] See "Framework for Cooperation Between UNRWA and the Government of the United States of America for 2011," U.S. Department of State, November 30, 2010, http://www.state.gov/documents/organization/154856.pdf.

[44] Colum Lynch, "UNESCO votes to admit Palestine; U.S. cuts off funding," *Washington Post*, October 31, 2011, http://www.washingtonpost.com/world/national-security/unesco-votes-to-admit-palestine-over-us-objections/2011/10/31/gIQAMleYZM_story.html.

[45] After Hamas formed the PA government in 2006 the United States passed P.L. 109-446, the Palestinian Anti-Terrorism Act of 2006, which restricted funding to any government that included Hamas. See Zanotti, "U.S. Foreign Aid to the Palestinians."

cannot support any government that consists of Hamas unless and until Hamas adopts the Quartet principles."[46]

Though it may tacitly accept the Quartet conditions at some point through rhetorical flexibility, Hamas is unlikely to explicitly accept these conditions in the foreseeable future. Recent comments by Hamas leader Khaled Meshal that Hamas is moving toward a common strategy with Fatah of "popular resistance" has fueled speculation that Hamas has made a strategic shift forgoing violence in its fight against Israel. Hamas has largely abided by a cease-fire with Israel since 2009 and calibrated its use of violence. There is considerable debate within Hamas's leadership on a range of issues, including recognizing Israel and the use of violence, but not on Hamas's right to use violence.[47]

Despite U.S. efforts to isolate Hamas, bolster Fatah, and oppose Palestinian reconciliation—and despite a nearly five-year Egyptian-Israeli blockade of Gaza—Hamas remains a potent and competent Palestinian political force. It has provided social services in Gaza and prevented a collapse of the government infrastructure in the face of intense economic and military efforts to dislodge it from power. Rather than weaken the movement, U.S. policy has helped strengthen its resolve and made more than 1.6 million Palestinians in Gaza increasingly dependent on Hamas. The dilemma remains that Hamas's ideology and use of violence against civilians is odious. Yet it is difficult to foresee any viable independent Palestinian state or lasting Israeli-Palestinian political agreement emerging without Hamas's acquiescence. Moreover, as the development of Gaza's health care sector indicates, Hamas's drive to build a record of governance feeds on influences that are often beyond the reach of the United States. Either as a movement, a political opposition, or part of a government, Hamas will remain a key actor and play a role shaping any future Palestinian political entity or state.

The ramifications for the United States are consequential, though difficult to quantify. U.S. policy has been premised on creating the conditions for a viable Palestinian state and mediating an Israeli-Palestinian agreement that will create that state. Should the Palestinian leadership and Mahmoud Abbas lose faith in U.S. efforts to create a Palestinian state, it would erode a key strategic rationale for the United States to serve as a regional mediator. It is less an issue of U.S. credibility, which is difficult to measure, than the erosion of the U.S. ability to shape Palestinian decisionmaking and outcomes. Other actors, who might have different agendas, will increasingly fill the void in providing assistance and counseling the Palestinians. This is already happening, and the trend is likely to continue.

---

[46] "Remarks with Italian Foreign Minister Franco Frattini," U.S. Department of State, May 5, 2011, http://www.state.gov/secretary/rm/2011/05/162581.htm.

[47] After Meshal's statement several Hamas leaders in Gaza announced that "armed resistance was a strategic option and the only way to liberate our land." See Harriet Sherwood, "Arab spring uprisings reveal rift in Hamas over conflict tactics," *The Guardian* (London), January 6, 2012, http://www.guardian.co.uk/world/2012/jan/06/arab-spring-hamas-rift-gaza.

For the Palestinians, funding cuts would not only affect direct budget support and security training, but also the PA's ability to provide social services. Funding cuts to the PA would almost certainly strengthen Hamas in the Hamas-Fatah power struggle, in part because Hamas has a better track record of providing social services outside of government frameworks. On the extreme end of the spectrum, funding cuts and estrangement between the United States and Palestinian leadership could over time erode the foundation of the PA and undermine chances for the creation of a viable Palestinian state.

U.S. policy has thus far sought to balance between broad support for Gaza's citizens and containing Hamas. Given the current trajectory of Palestinian and regional trends, the U.S. government will increasingly find itself facing difficult choices in pursuing ways that preserve its leverage while promoting U.S. interests.

www.ingramcontent.com/pod-product-compliance
Ingram Content Group UK Ltd.
Pitfield, Milton Keynes, MK11 3LW, UK
UKHW051418150926
475561UK00005B/237